Swim Your Ass Off!

A Fun & Easy Guide to Swimming for Weight Loss,
Health, and Blood Sugar Control

No Olympic Pool Needed!

Kevin John Grabian

Swim Your Ass Off
© 2025 Kevin John Grabian
All Rights Reserved.

No part of this book may be reproduced, stored in a retrieval system, or transmitted in any form or by any means—electronic, mechanical, photocopying, recording, or otherwise—without prior written permission from the author, except for brief quotations in a review or reference.

Disclaimer

This book is for informational and educational purposes only. The author and publisher are not responsible for any injuries or damages resulting from the application of the techniques or recommendations in this book. Always consult a qualified professional before beginning any new fitness program.

ISBN: 979-8-218-63549-7

Published by Kevin John Grabian

Contents

Introduction..…..…....1

Part I: Getting Started with Swimming for Fitness

Ch 1: Why Swimming is the Best Exercise for You…......5

Ch 2: Setting Yourself Up for Success...................…....11

Ch 3: Mastering the Basics – Strokes and Techniques...19

Part II: Building Your Swimming Workout Plan

Ch 4: Creating a Swim Workout – No Matter Your Pool Size..…...31

Ch 5: How to Build Endurance & Burn Fat............…...47

Part III: The Diet and Lifestyle Changes That Made the Difference

Ch 6: Nutrition Plan for Weight Loss and Blood Sugar Control..................................…......................61

Ch 7: Balancing Swimming with Other Healthy Habits..65

The Swim Your ASS Off Challenge!........................71

Introduction

I get it. You want to lose weight, get in shape, and feel better—but everything you've tried so far has either been too hard on your body, too complicated, or just plain boring. Maybe you've struggled with injuries, chronic pain, or health issues that make traditional workouts miserable. Maybe you've started a fitness routine a dozen times, only to quit when motivation fades. I've been there.

My Story: From Pain to Progress

For years, I struggled with plantar fasciitis. The pain was relentless, but I pushed through—until one day, I partially tore my plantar fascia. The pain was unbearable. Walking became a challenge, let alone exercising. I was nearly crippled by the injury and had to stop working out altogether. Every step felt like I was walking on broken glass, and the frustration of being sidelined only made things worse.

At the same time, I was dealing with severe shoulder pain and a limited range of motion. Lifting weights was out of the question, and even simple daily activities became difficult. The combination of these injuries left me feeling defeated, out of shape, and uncertain about how to regain my health.

Then came the wake-up call: after battling a severe case of COVID, I was diagnosed with diabetes. My blood sugar was climbing, and I knew I had to make a change. But how could I exercise when my body felt like it was working against me?

That's when I found swimming. Not Olympic-style laps in a giant pool, but real, practical, everyday swimming—even in small spaces. I started at my local fitness center in a pool that's only 26 feet long. In the summer, I used my own tiny 15-foot backyard pool with a simple swimming tether. No excuses, no fancy equipment—just water, movement, and commitment. And guess what? It worked.

I lost 40 pounds. I gained energy. My blood sugar levels stabilized. My body, once wrecked with pain, started to feel strong again. And I did it all without pounding the pavement or lifting heavy weights.

This book isn't about becoming an elite swimmer. It's not about perfection. It's about getting in the water and moving your body in a way that works for you. Whether you have access to a large pool or just a small backyard setup, you can swim your way to better health—no matter where you're starting from.

So, if you're tired of fitness routines that leave you sore, frustrated, and unmotivated, this guide is for you. No gimmicks, no fluff—just a simple, effective way to lose weight, get fit, and feel amazing.

It's time to **swim your ASS off**.   Let's go!

Part I: Getting Started with Swimming for Fitness

Ch 1: Why Swimming is the Best Exercise for You

Key Benefits of Swimming for Fitness:

- Low impact on joints – Perfect for injury prevention & recovery.
- Improves cardiovascular health – Strengthens the heart & lungs.
- Full-body engagement – No muscle group is left behind.
- Boosts flexibility & mobility – The water's resistance improves range of motion.
- Enhances endurance – Builds stamina without excessive wear and tear.

With the right techniques and consistency, swimming can transform your body by sculpting lean muscles and accelerating fat loss. Whether you're looking to get stronger, leaner, or improve endurance, the pool offers a versatile and effective workout solution.

Low-Impact Benefits for Injuries and Joint Pain

Everyone has been there—just getting into the groove of a new fitness regimen, and then *bam*, injury. You stop working out to heal, but sometimes the injury never fully goes away. All that time away from your routine drains your motivation. By the time you're ready to start again, you just don't feel it anymore.

This cycle repeats for so many people who are simply trying to get in shape. No matter your situation—whether you're currently pain-free, dealing with limited mobility due to an injury, or recovering but afraid of re-injury—swimming is the answer. It's the total-body workout you've been looking for. The benefits are numerous: increased flexibility, mobility, strength, endurance, and reduced body fat. And the best part? You can achieve all of this without pain!

Full-Body Workout: Cardio + Strength in One

After wrapping up a swim session, you'll feel it *everywhere*. The cardio aspect keeps your heart rate up and burns calories, while your muscles—everything from your legs and back to your abs, shoulders, and chest—engage in a full workout. You might even feel a little sore at first, but don't worry—that's the *good* kind of soreness. It's a sign that your muscles are strengthening and growing, not the kind of pain that signals injury.

Another great perk? Many people find that their chronic joint pain—whether in the knees, ankles, or shoulders—dramatically improves after regular swimming sessions. And the effects linger long after you get out of the water.

Ideal for Diabetics and Those Struggling with Weight Loss

When I was diagnosed with diabetes, I got a continuous glucose monitor as soon as I could. What I learned was eye-opening! Even after eating a carb-heavy meal, if I went swimming soon after, my blood sugar remained within my target range.

As I swam, I could literally *watch* my glucose levels drop in real time. My body responded just like a non-diabetic's: my blood sugar would start to rise after eating, but then I'd see a sharp downward curve as soon as I hit the pool. It would stabilize at a healthy level and stay there.

This has been a game-changer for me in two ways:

1. **Motivation** – I know that if I swim after a meal, it will help regulate my blood sugar, so I make sure to get to the pool.

2. **Mindful Eating** – While I can "get away" with more carbs if I swim, it has also made me more conscious of what I eat.

Swimming has given me control over my body in a way no other workout ever has. And it can do the same for you.

Overcoming Common Fears (Not Being a Strong Swimmer, Feeling Self-Conscious, etc.)

Maybe you consider yourself a strong swimmer, or maybe you feel like you sink like a rock. No matter your skill level, you can build an exercise routine that works for you and helps you get fit.

If you don't know how to swim at all, don't worry—you're not alone! Many fitness centers offer adult swim classes that can teach you the basics. You can also learn on your own with guidance from online resources or with the help of a friend. It's okay if you're not comfortable in the water yet; the important thing is to start. If necessary, wear a snug-fitting life jacket designed for water sports until you gain confidence.

If you haven't been swimming in a long time, take it easy at first. **DO NOT** try to swim across a deep 25-meter pool on your first day! Instead, start at the edge, swim a short distance, then swim back. Gradually build up your stamina and technique.

For those who already swim somewhat regularly, great job! You can refine your technique and create a structured fitness routine that challenges you.

No matter where you are on this journey, it's normal to feel self-conscious at first. But don't let that hold you back! The more you get in the water, the more those feelings will fade. I remember feeling awkward when I first started using my gym's small aerobics pool for swimming exercises. People looked at me like I was crazy! But over time, they got used to it. Eventually, when gym staff gave tours, they would even point me out as an example of how the pool could be used for more than just aerobics.

The key is to **show up, keep going, and focus on your progress.** Your confidence will grow with each swim!

Creating a Simple Swimming Routine That Fits into Your Life

Whether you have limited time for fitness or a more flexible schedule (lucky you!), you can create a solid swimming plan that delivers results. The key is consistency and finding a routine that works for you.

Personally, I aim to swim at least three times per week. In the summer, I often swim daily—mainly because I have a pool in my yard, so I have no excuse not to! But you don't need a backyard pool to build a habit. Start with just **one swim per week** and gradually increase as you become more comfortable.

The biggest challenge isn't the workout itself—it's showing up. **Don't make excuses not to go!** In fact, once you experience the benefits of swimming as exercise, you'll probably start making excuses **to** go for a swim. Stick with it, and soon it will become a natural (and enjoyable) part of your routine.

Ch 2: Setting Yourself Up for Success

Finding a Local Pool or Using What You Have

Everyone will have different swimming options available to them. If you live in an area with cold winters, your swimming spot may change throughout the year. That's okay—be flexible and just focus on getting in the water!

There are many options for swimming. Here are a few places that you may need to seek out in your area to get your swimming journey started. None of these are necessarily better than the others; each has its benefits and drawbacks. Let's explore your options:

Large Swimming Pools

An Olympic-size pool is 50 meters long—talk about intimidating! Many pools at larger fitness centers are 25 meters long and divided into swimming lanes with floating rope dividers. These pools are typically heated to around 78°F and can be quite deep, with no shallow sections. If you aren't a strong swimmer or can't swim at all, there are better options for you! If this is your only option, consider wearing a life jacket until you feel more comfortable. You don't need to swim the entire length at once—start at the edge, swim out a bit, and return. Over time, your stamina and form will improve.

Fitness or Aerobic Pools

Many smaller fitness centers often have small pools, usually around 25 feet in length and no deeper than 4 feet 6 inches—good news if you can't swim yet! Some are even heated slightly higher than larger pools and may use saltwater for additional benefits. Though they may seem too small for a good workout, they are actually perfect for swimming exercises, even when shared with others.

Public Pools

Public pools, often open only in the summer in northern areas, often have designated swimming areas suitable for exercise. Visiting early in the morning can help you avoid busy times and allow for a more comfortable workout.

Hotel Pools

With a length of at least 25 feet, hotel pools offer a perfect space for exercise. While some may have a deeper end, they usually include a shallow section to start in. Hotel pools are often less crowded, except during youth sports tournaments or peak travel seasons.

Home Pools

Home pools come in a variety of shapes and sizes, from in-ground to above-ground, square to oblong. Depths vary, but many are less than 5 feet deep. Even a small home pool (10 feet across) can be used for exercise swimming! The benefits of smaller pools are that they require fewer chemicals to maintain and are more affordable.

Swim Spa Pools

These pools resemble hot tubs but include a powerful water current to swim against, simulating the experience of swimming in a river. They are usually shallow enough to stand in and often include seating and jacuzzi jets for post-swim relaxation.

Natural Bodies of Water

Lakes, rivers, and ponds can all be used for exercise swimming, but safety precautions are essential. I follow a strict rule: I don't swim in open water without some form of flotation (such as a towable flotation device) unless I know for certain that I can stand up in the water. Wearing a life jacket is a great option—and yes, you can still swim in one!

No matter what your situation is, there's always a way to get into the water and start swimming. Find what works best for you and dive in!

Gear You Actually Need (Minimalist Approach)

To get started with swimming as an exercise, you'll need a few essential items to make your workout comfortable and effective. Some of these items are optional, depending on your situation. Don't worry about how you look—this isn't a fashion show! Focus on getting in the water and swimming.

Swimwear

For exercise swimming, your swimwear shouldn't be too baggy. Avoid trunks that extend past your knees if possible. Any style of swimwear can work, but athletic swimwear is ideal. These suits, usually a polyester-spandex blend, fit snugly and reduce drag in the water, making swimming easier and more efficient.

Goggles

A good pair of swim goggles is absolutely necessary. They come in various eye-cup styles and sizes. I prefer the middle eye-socket fit because it's comfortable and provides a great seal. If you have poor vision, consider goggles with prescription lenses so you don't lose your bearings in the pool. Also, grab some anti-fog spray to maintain visibility during your swims.

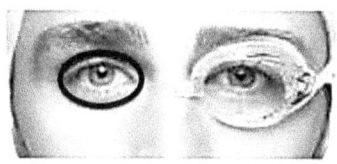

Inner Eye Fit: low profile, rests snuggly in the eye socket

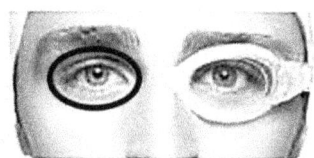

Middle Eye Fit: comfortable fit, rests within the eye orbital but not so tight within the eye socket

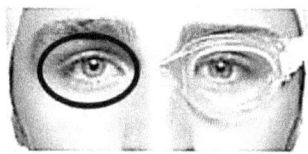

Outer Eye Fit: most universal fit for different face shapes, fits outside the eye socket

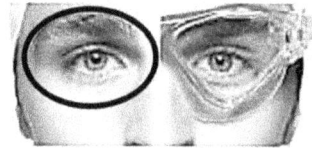

Mask Fit: very comfortable fit well outside eye orbital, not as low profile as other options

Ear Plugs

Swimming earplugs are a must if you plan to make swimming a regular workout. They keep your inner ear dry and prevent painful ear infections—I learned this the hard way! Choose earplugs designed for swimming, as foam earplugs made for noise reduction will expand and slide out of your ears in the water.

Shampoo and Conditioner

If you swim in a chlorinated pool, invest in a good swimmer's shampoo and conditioner to protect your hair. Some swimmers prefer to use a swim cap to minimize chlorine exposure—this is definitely an option!

Waterproof Headphones

Music can make workouts more enjoyable, but regular speakers won't work underwater. That's where waterproof bone-conduction headphones come in. These headphones rest on your temples and transmit sound through bone conduction, allowing you to hear music clearly while swimming. Look for models with built-in MP3 storage, as Bluetooth won't work underwater.

Swimming Tether

If you're using a small pool, consider a swimming tether. This elastic leash attaches to a fixed point (like a handrail or deck) and clips around your waist, allowing you to swim in place. It's great for getting a full workout even in limited space. I always keep one in my gym bag in case the pool is crowded. A snorkel can also be useful with a tether, letting you breathe easily while focusing on your form. This setup is also perfect for travel if you're staying at a hotel with a small pool.

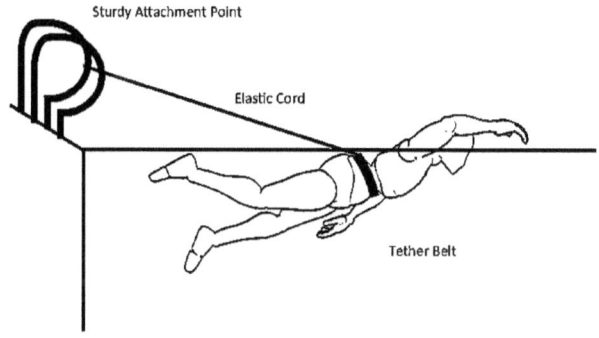

Swimming Tether

Mesh Bag

A small mesh bag is perfect for carrying wet towels and swimwear home after your workout. It dries quickly and keeps your gym bag from getting soggy. I also store my swimming tether in a separate mesh bag—after using it, I just hang the whole bag to dry in my shower at home!

Ch 3: Mastering the Basics – Strokes and Techniques

Swimming Strokes You Need to Know

There are many different ways to swim, and guess what? They can all be used for exercise! I like to switch up my swimming style during workouts to engage different muscle groups, so try to get proficient at a few of these strokes. One important note about breathing: If you are doing a stroke where your head is submerged, exhale slowly through your nose as you complete the motion. Then, when you pop your head or mouth out for a breath, take a quick inhale through your mouth. Exhaling through the nose and inhaling through the mouth will help prevent water from going up your nose!

Doggy Paddle

That's right—this beginner swimming method can be used for exercise! Try doggy paddling for 20 minutes and tell me you didn't get a workout. This basic stroke is useful for both beginners and experts. If you cannot swim and are wearing a life jacket, this is the stroke to start with. Focus on making your hands into scoops (keep your fingers together) and alternately scooping left and right with your arms. While doing this, kick your feet at a comfortable pace, trying to point your toes back. Your head and face should remain out of the water while swimming in this style.

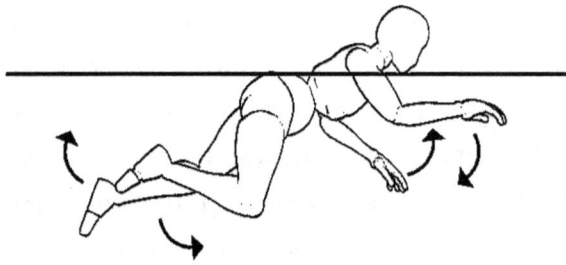

Doggy Paddle

Side Stroke

This stroke is a great next step for those advancing from the doggy paddle and an excellent way for advanced swimmers to engage different muscle groups. To perform the side stroke, lie on your side, outstretch your hands, and scoop them back alternately while using a scissor kick with your feet. This stroke is helpful as a lifesaving technique and is often used in long-distance swimming events. Swimmers can switch which side they have facing forward to target different muscle groups.

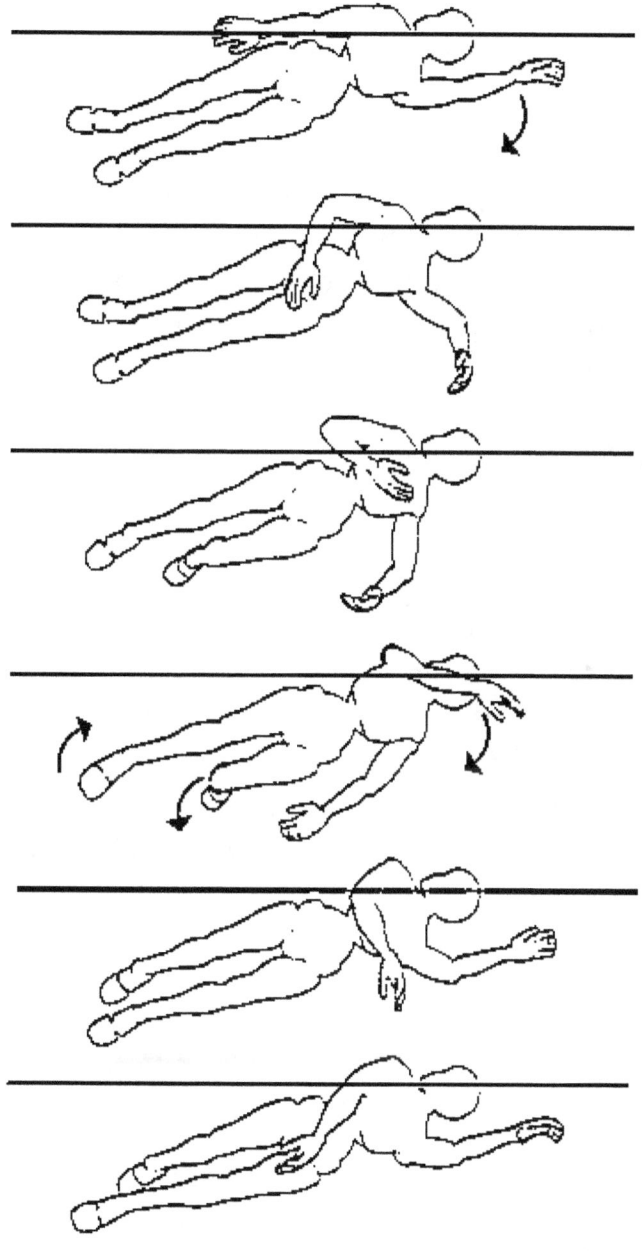

Side Stroke

Modified Breaststroke

For this stroke, reach out in front with both hands while submerging your head. Then, turn your hands outward and pull them back and to the sides. A standard breaststroke has a short pull, but in this modified version for exercise, keep your hands wide and pull all the way back until your arms form a "T" with your body. From this position, with your hands facing back towards your feet, quickly continue the stroke back until your hands almost touch your legs. This will engage your chest and shoulder muscles.

You can choose to kick, using frog, flutter, or scissor kicking, or focus solely on your upper body. As you reach the point of the stroke where your arms are out like a "T", be sure to give it a little extra effort for the final push as your hands come down to your legs. This helps lift your head out of the water for a breath. Be sure to exhale as your arms go through the pulling motion of the stroke and inhale as your head pops out of the water.

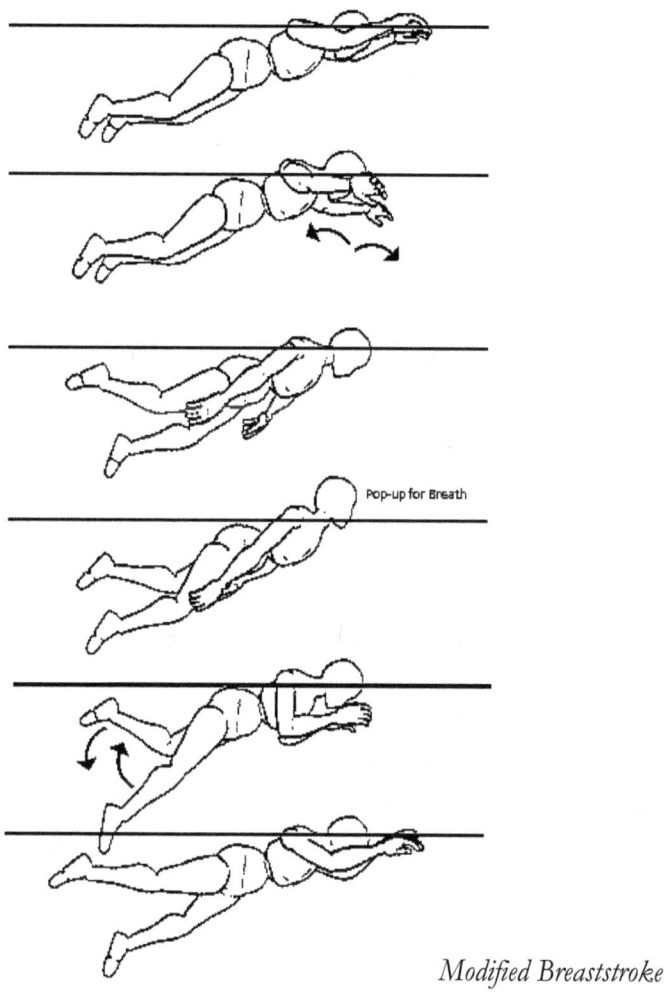

Modified Breaststroke

Legs Only

This stroke uses a flotation device called a kickboard. Hold the kickboard in front of you with outstretched arms, hands placed at the front edge of the board, and kick your legs alternately back and forth. Kick from your hips, extending your legs and avoiding any bit of knee bending. Try to point your toes straight behind you, turned slightly inside, to maximize efficiency.

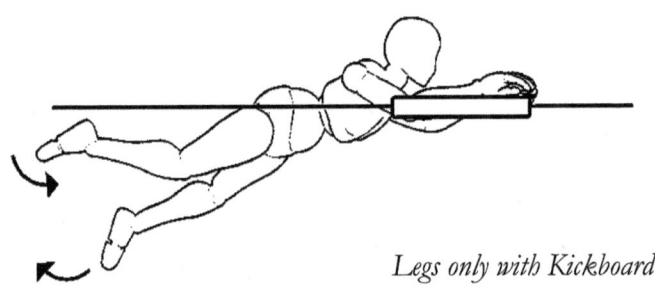

Legs only with Kickboard

Front Crawl or Freestyle

Freestyle is the fastest stroke and should be on your list to master. Lie face down, alternately bringing one arm up over your head and scooping the water in front of you, pulling back as the other arm begins its motion. While moving your arms, flutter kick your legs at a slightly faster pace than your arm strokes.

While you can keep your head above water, it's more efficient to submerge it between breaths. Keep your head facing downward and slightly forward. Exhale while your head is underwater so you're ready to inhale when needed. To breathe, tilt your body and head opposite the reaching arm, taking a quick breath from the corner of your mouth that is facing upward.

If you are reaching forward with your left arm, tilt your head to the right for a breath. This technique may take practice but will soon feel natural.

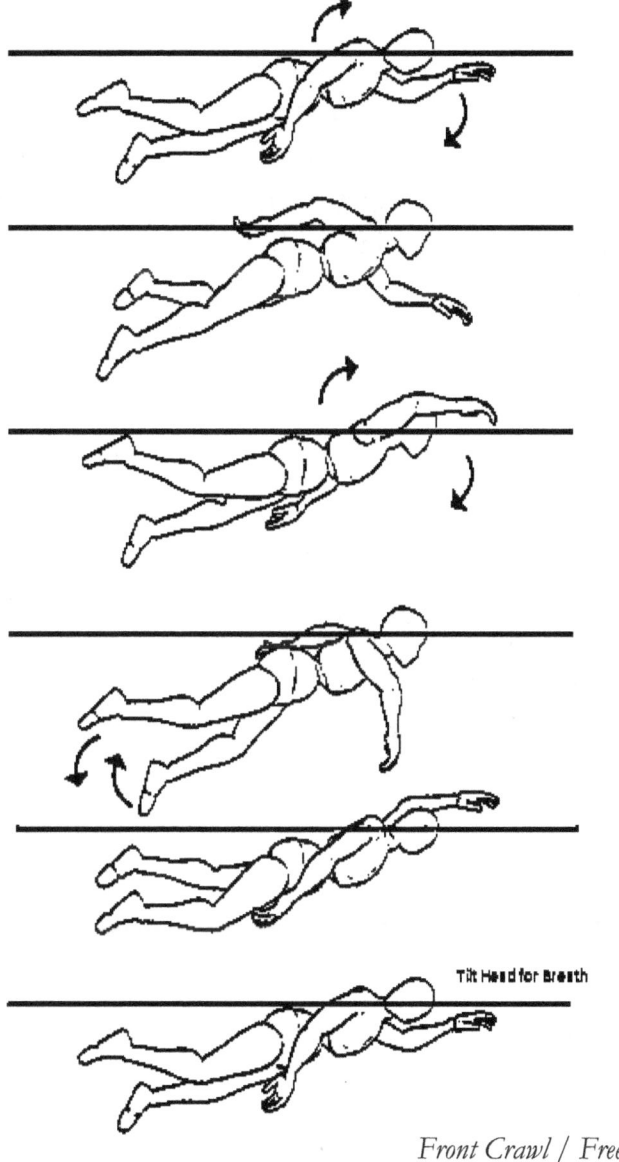

Front Crawl / Freestyle

Backstroke

For shoulder mobility, try the backstroke. Lie on your back and rotate one arm up and over your head, keeping the motion tight so that your arm brushes your ear. As one hand enters the water, the other arm should be rising from the opposite direction. As your front arm enters the water, scoop with your palm facing upward and pull through. Keep the rotation tight, aiming to brush your leg as you finish the stroke.

While your arms do most of the work, you'll need to flutter kick to stay horizontal. Take a deep breath before starting, exhaling through your nose if your head submerges slightly. Take quick breaths when your mouth clears the water using an occasional explosive stroke from one arm. Keep your eyes on the ceiling and carefully feel for the wall as you approach the end of your lane.

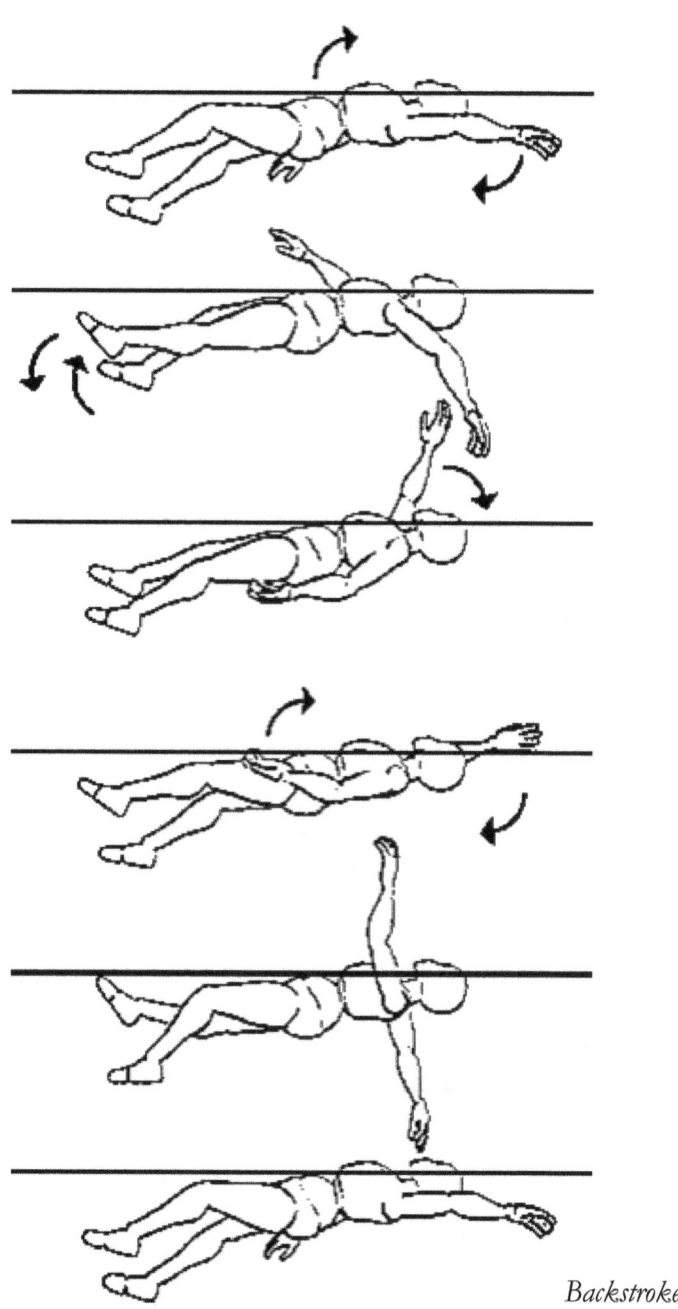

Backstroke

Underwater Push-Off

For a full-body workout, incorporate explosive leg movement. Exhale and use your hands to push yourself downward. Firmly plant your feet against the pool wall and push off explosively, gliding parallel to the bottom. Keep your head down and your hands outstretched to reduce drag. Aim to propel yourself across a 25-foot pool with one push-off. If you don't make it across, complete a full "T" breaststroke to reach the opposite end before surfacing.

This method is suitable only for in-ground pools or sturdy above-ground pools. Do not attempt to kick off from the side of a standard above-ground pool, as it may cause damage!

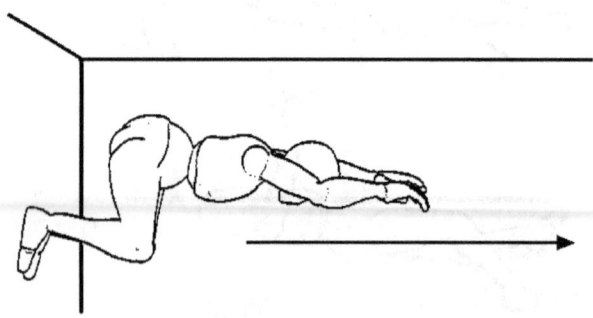

Underwater Push-Off

By practicing these strokes, you'll build endurance, improve technique, and get a great workout in the pool!

If you're unsure how to improve your technique for these swimming methods, watching instructional videos online can be incredibly helpful. To take it a step further, try recording yourself swimming or ask a friend to film you. Then, compare your footage to professional demonstrations to spot areas for improvement. This method helped me go from an average swimmer to a really strong one in just a few weeks!

Part II: Building Your Swimming Workout Plan

Ch 4: Creating a Swim Workout – No Matter Your Pool Size

Interval training for a tiny pool (using a tether for resistance)

If all you have access to is a small pool, or your local pool is too crowded for laps, don't worry! A swimming tether can help you get an effective workout in almost any space. These routines are perfect if you have access to an endless lap "Swim Spa" style pool.

To set up, secure one end of the tether to a sturdy structure like a pool railing, towel hook, or deck post. At home, I attach mine to a solid post on my wooden deck, which extends to the edge of my 15-foot pool. I also shorten the tether slightly to ensure that when fully stretched, I remain centered in the pool and don't hit the opposite side.

Once the belt is secured around your waist and tightened, you're ready to begin. Simply stretch out and start swimming, pulling against the tether's resistance. The harder you swim, the more resistance you'll feel, making for a great workout!

Since you won't be swimming laps, this workout focuses on timed intervals. Use an interval timing app on your phone, placing it somewhere safe, but close enough so that you can hear the timer go off. I enjoy wearing waterproof bone conduction headphones, using songs as a timing source. Each song is around 3 minutes long.

Beginner Tether Routine

Start by facing away from the tether anchor point and begin with a doggy paddle. If that's too difficult, try running in place against the tether's resistance. Need more of a challenge? Shorten the tether for added resistance.

- **3 minutes** – Doggy Paddle

- **3 minutes** – Legs Only (using a kickboard)

- **3 minutes** – Side Stroke

- **3 minutes** – Running in place against the tether

- **Repeat**

Try completing this routine twice, increasing to three of four rounds as you build endurance.

Intermediate Tether Routine

Once you're comfortable with the beginner routine, level up with this workout. Don't worry if you can't complete it all at first—just keep moving and do what you can!

- **4 minutes** – Side Stroke
- **4 minutes** – Legs Only (using a kickboard)
- **4 minutes** – Front Crawl
- **4 minutes** – Modified Breaststroke
- **Repeat**

Aim for two full rounds, working your way up to three or four rounds before progressing to the advanced routine.

Advanced Tether Routine

For a full-body, high-intensity workout, this routine will push your limits. If you want to focus on form, consider wearing a snorkel to avoid breathing interruptions.

- **5 minutes** – Front Crawl (casual intensity)
- **5 minutes** – Modified Breaststroke
- **5 minutes** – Front Crawl (medium intensity)
- **5 minutes** – Modified Breaststroke
- **5 minutes** – Front Crawl (high intensity)
- **5 minutes** – Backstroke

During the final high-intensity front crawl, the tether should be fully stretched, bringing you close to the opposite end of the pool. For the backstroke, rotate the belt so the tether is positioned in the front for proper resistance.

Swimming in natural bodies of water

Swimming in natural bodies of water, such as ponds, lakes, or rivers, can be a great alternative to pool swimming, but extra caution is necessary. Never attempt to swim in fast-moving water, regardless of your skill level, as currents can be unpredictable and dangerous. Beginners should avoid swimming in water that is over their heads, as depth can be difficult to gauge. Always take extreme precautions, wear a flotation device, and never swim alone.

Water temperature is another important factor to consider. Experts recommend a minimum water temperature of 78°F for safe swimming. If the water is colder, a wetsuit can help retain body heat and make swimming more comfortable. Additionally, swimmers should be aware of other potential dangers, such as tidal changes, rip currents, boating traffic, and subsurface hazards like sharp rocks or stumps. Weather conditions can also pose significant risks, so it's essential to stay informed and avoid swimming if conditions seem unsafe. If you have any doubts about the safety of the water, it's best to stay on shore.

One of my favorite places to swim is at a small campground we visit each year. The designated swimming area minimizes boat traffic, and the sandy bottom has a gradual drop-off, making it easy to wade out without sudden depth changes. I usually swim only in areas I have scouted beforehand, ensuring I can touch the bottom if needed. If I ever swim in water where I can't touch or am uncertain about the depth, I always have a flotation device for added safety.

Unlike pools, natural bodies of water are not ideal for traditional lap swimming, so a time-based approach works best for workouts. It's important to stay within the area you've identified as safe. If you want to create a designated swim zone, you can make your own swim buoys by:

1. Tying a piece of clothesline or similar rope to a small milk jug filled with sand and re-capped. This will serve as an anchor.
2. At the other end of the rope, attach an empty, sealed milk jug to act as a buoy.
3. Leave a bit of extra rope at this end, allowing you to secure your kickboard when not in use.

For workouts in open water, follow the routines outlined in the "Interval Training for a Tiny Pool" section. Many of the strokes included in these circuits can be performed while wearing a life jacket. Another great option, even for experienced swimmers, is to use a swimmer's safety float. These brightly colored devices attach to a belt and are towed behind you, making you more visible while also providing a resting aid if needed.

Swimming in natural bodies of water can be a fantastic way to stay active and enjoy the outdoors, but safety should always come first. By taking proper precautions, being aware of potential hazards, and staying within designated safe areas, you can make open water swimming a fun and rewarding experience.

Workout routines for medium sized pools

The following workouts are designed for pools that are at least 20 feet in length. These routines are primarily lap-based rather than timed intervals, but you can easily use a timer instead of counting laps. Get creative! I personally follow these routines in the 26-foot pool at my local fitness center.

For reference, the term "lap" in this section refers to swimming one length of the pool—from one end to the other. A round trip (down and back) counts as two laps.

Beginner Medium Pool Routine

If you're not a strong swimmer, ensure you can touch the bottom for the entire length of the pool. While this usually isn't an issue in medium-sized pools, check beforehand. If you can't touch the bottom at any point, consider wearing a flotation device or avoiding deeper areas.

If you're returning to swimming after a long break, this is a great routine to start with:

- **10 laps** – Doggy Paddle

- **8 laps** – Legs Only (using a kickboard)

- **6 laps** – Side Stroke

- **Repeat**

Your initial goal is to complete this circuit twice. As your stamina and technique improve, aim for three or more rounds. To challenge yourself, time one complete circuit and try to beat your record!

Intermediate Medium Pool Routine

Once you're ready to advance beyond the beginner routine, try this circuit. If you struggle to complete all the laps, don't worry—just keep moving! If needed, switch to an easier stroke temporarily before resuming the routine.

- **10 laps** – Side Stroke
- **8 laps** – Legs Only (using a kickboard)
- **6 laps** – Front Crawl (casual intensity)
- **4 laps** – Modified Breaststroke
- **2 laps** – Front Crawl (medium intensity)
- **Repeat**

Start by completing this circuit once and recording your time. During your next session, try to improve your time. Once you feel confident, work toward completing at least two full rounds—or more!

Advanced Medium Pool Routine

If you've mastered the beginner and intermediate routines, it's time to level up! This high-intensity routine is designed for swimmers with good form and endurance.

This is my go-to workout:

- **10 laps** – Front Crawl (casual intensity)
- **10 laps** – Front Crawl (medium intensity)
- **10 laps** – Modified Breaststroke
- **10 laps** – Underwater Push-off (down)
    - Backstroke (on the return lap)
- **12 laps** – Front Crawl (high intensity)
- **Repeat**

In a 26-foot pool, completing one full circuit of this routine equals approximately a **quarter mile!** I like to push myself through two rounds of this workout completing a **half mile of swimming,** ramping up the effort in the final laps.

For added variety—if your pool is deep enough—consider incorporating kickflips at the turnaround points during your front crawl segments.

Using large pools for exercise

Your local fitness center may not have anything smaller than a 25-meter (or even an Olympic size) pool. That's ok! Don't be intimidated. I have adjusted the different workout circuits for both a standard Olympic size pool (50-meters) and a common large pool found at fitness centers (25-meters), making adjustments to avoid laps that are not complete.

Do not use these larger pools if you aren't a strong swimmer unless you wear a flotation device! These pools are generally deeper, and you may not be able to touch the bottom. If you are a beginner, find a shallow pool until you have at least a beginner level of swimming skills.

Beginner Large Pool Routine

If you're using a 25-meter pool:

- **4 laps** – Doggy Paddle
- **2 laps** – Legs Only (using a kickboard)
- **2 laps** – Side Stroke
- **Repeat**

If you're using a 50-meter pool:

- **2 laps** – Doggy Paddle
- **1 lap** – Legs Only (using a kickboard)
- **1 lap** – Side Stroke
- **Repeat**

When using large pools, stay within a distance from the edge that feels safe and comfortable for you, especially when starting out. Go out a short distance and turn around the first few times. Do this until you feel confident in making it all the way across. Then, work on hitting the lap goals in these circuits!

Intermediate Large Pool Routine

If you're using a 25-meter pool:

- **4 laps** – Side Stroke
- **2 laps** – Legs Only (using a kickboard)
- **1 lap** – Front Crawl (casual intensity)
- **1 lap** – Modified Breaststroke
- **1 lap** – Front Crawl (medium intensity)
- **Repeat**

If you're using a 50-meter pool:

- **1 lap** – Side Stroke
- **1 lap** – Legs Only (using a kickboard)
- **1 lap** – Front Crawl (casual intensity)
- **1 lap** – Modified Breaststroke
- **1 lap** – Front Crawl (medium intensity)
- **Repeat**

Time yourself for a full circuit then try and shave a little time off each time you visit the pool!

Advanced Large Pool Routine

If you're using a 25-meter pool:

- **4 laps** – Front Crawl (casual intensity)
- **2 laps** – Front Crawl (medium intensity)
- **4 laps** – Modified Breaststroke
- **1 lap** – Underwater Push-off (down as far as you can go), then Side Stroke
- **1 lap** – Backstroke
- **4 laps** – Front Crawl (high intensity)
- **Repeat**

If you're using a 50-meter pool:

- **2 laps** – Front Crawl (casual intensity)
- **1 lap** – Front Crawl (medium intensity)
- **2 laps** – Modified Breaststroke
- **1 lap** – Underwater Push-off (down as far as you can go), then Backstroke
- **2 laps** – Front Crawl (high intensity)
- **Repeat**

Ch 5: How to Build Endurance & Burn Fat

Start Small and Build

The first time you step into the pool for your new workout routine, take a moment to pause. This is the beginning of your journey toward a healthier version of yourself. That water will become a symbol of your progress. Soon, the smell of chlorine will remind you of dedication and growth. Savor this moment and commit to the path ahead.

Let's be honest—your first swimming session probably won't go perfectly. If you're anything like me, you'll spend more time than expected adjusting your goggles, re-tying your swim trunks, trying to remember what lap you were on, and, inevitably, swallowing a bit of pool water. That's okay! A less-than-perfect swim is still far better than not getting in the water at all.

Your main goal for the first session is simple: get in and gauge where you're at. Can you complete basic swimming strokes? Practice them and see how they feel. How long can you hold your breath while swimming? When I started, I needed to breathe with nearly every stroke. Now, I can easily swim the full length of a 26-foot pool without taking a breath. These are the small improvements you'll work toward over time.

If you can't complete 10 laps right away, that's fine. Do what you can today, then aim for just one more lap next time. Then one more after that. Before you know it, 10 laps will feel effortless, and you'll be wondering how you ever struggled with it.

As your endurance builds, don't let yourself get too comfortable. Instead of resting when things start to feel easier, challenge yourself. Swim faster, hold your breath longer, or refine your strokes to become more efficient. Increase your lap count, push to beat your best time, and switch up your strokes—do whatever it takes to keep improving.

One important thing: never compare yourself to others in the pool. There will always be someone swimming faster, farther, or more gracefully. That doesn't matter. You're not trying to beat them. The only person you need to beat is the version of yourself from your last swim session.

When I started, I could barely complete 10 laps in a 26-foot pool, flailing and gasping for air by the end. Now, I swim 52 laps (a **half mile**) regularly with ease. I push myself to keep my heart rate up, and it feels incredible. You'll be amazed at how far you can go—just take it one lap at a time.

Breathing Tips for Endurance

Breathing efficiently while swimming is essential for endurance. I've already mentioned a few fundamental techniques, such as exhaling through your nose underwater, taking a quick but deep breath at the surface, and timing your inhale by turning your head with the front crawl. Now, let's explore additional breathing methods that can help you swim longer with less fatigue.

Establishing an Effective Breathing Rhythm

To breathe efficiently while swimming, follow these steps:

1. Keep your head aligned with your body – Look downward to maintain a natural body position.

2. Time your inhale with your stroke – As your arm moves forward, rotate your head just enough to get a breath without disrupting your form.

3. Exhale fully underwater – Release air smoothly through your nose or mouth before turning your head to inhale.

4. Develop a breathing pattern – Beginners may start by breathing every three strokes, while more experienced swimmers may adjust based on comfort and endurance.

5. Breathe naturally – Avoid holding your breath; instead, maintain a steady cycle of inhaling and exhaling.

As you practice, these techniques will become second nature, making it easier to swim for extended periods without tiring.

Building Endurance with Advanced Breathing Drills

Once you've mastered the basics, challenge yourself with these breathing exercises to improve lung capacity and swimming efficiency:

- Increase breath-holding intervals – Start by breathing every four or five strokes to push your lung capacity. Over time, work up to every six or seven strokes for short distances.

- Alternate breathing sides – Switching between left and right breathing in each lap promotes balanced muscle development and prevents overuse on one side.

- - Focus on single-side breathing – Strengthen lung capacity by practicing a full lap breathing only on your non-dominant side.

- Adapt your breathing to different strokes:

  - Freestyle: Breathe every 2–3 strokes to maintain rhythm.

  - Backstroke: Inhale as one arm extends above the water. I inhale as my right arm extends out and exhale when my left arm comes out of the water.

  - Breaststroke: Inhale as your head rises naturally during the stroke.

- Try rhythmic breathing – Inhale on one side and exhale smoothly to the opposite side as you swim. This technique can help reduce drag and improve speed, especially for competitive swimmers.

By practicing these drills, you'll train your body to use oxygen more efficiently, helping you swim longer with less effort. You'll develop greater efficiency, stamina, and confidence in the water. With consistent practice, proper breathing will feel effortless, allowing you to focus on endurance and technique.

Swimming to Build Muscle, Burn Fat

Swimming is one of the most effective full-body workouts, combining muscle strengthening and fat burning while being gentle on the joints. Whether you're looking to tone your muscles, shed excess weight, or boost endurance, swimming provides a dynamic and low-impact way to reach your fitness goals.

Calories Burned & Fat Loss in Swimming

Swimming engages multiple muscle groups at once, making it a high-calorie-burning activity. The number of calories burned depends on factors like stroke type, intensity, and body weight. Here's a general estimate of calories burned per hour while swimming vigorously:

- Freestyle (moderate effort): 500–600 calories

- Freestyle (vigorous effort): 700–900 calories

- Breaststroke: 600–750 calories

- Backstroke: 400–500 calories

To maximize fat burning, aim to keep your heart rate in the fat-burning zone (around 60–70% of your max heart rate). A mix of steady-state swimming and high-intensity intervals will help you achieve this.

Fat-Burning Swimming Tips: Swim continuously for at least 30–45 minutes to keep your body in fat-burning mode. Use interval training – alternate between fast-paced sprints and slower recovery laps to boost metabolism. Incorporate different strokes – switching between strokes keeps the workout dynamic and engages more muscles.

Building Muscle Through Swimming

Swimming naturally builds lean, strong muscles because the water provides constant resistance. Unlike weightlifting, where resistance comes from external weights, water resistance works against every movement you make, forcing your muscles to engage more deeply.

Major Muscle Groups Activated in Swimming

Upper Body:

1. Arms & Shoulders – Strokes like freestyle, breaststroke, and backstroke work the biceps, triceps, and deltoids.

2. Chest – The motion from the modified breaststroke will not only work the shoulders but will also engage the pectoral muscles.

3. Back & Lats – The pulling motion strengthens the latissimus dorsi and trapezius.

Core & Torso:

4. Abdominals & Obliques – Rotational movements during front crawl and backstroke help develop a strong core.

5. Lower Back – Keeping the body aligned in the water strengthens spinal stabilizers.

Lower Body:

6. Legs & Glutes – Kicking movements in all strokes work the quadriceps, hamstrings, calves, and glutes.

7. Hips & Inner Thighs – The frog kick in breaststroke targets the adductors and abductors.

Since water supports the body, swimming allows for muscle growth without excessive strain on the joints, making it an excellent alternative to weight training.

Maximizing Muscle Growth & Fat Burn in the Pool

To increase muscle definition and fat loss, try these swimming techniques:

1. Interval Training for Fat Loss & Endurance

    - Swim fast sprints for 30–60 seconds, then recover with an easy swim for 30 seconds.
    - Repeat this for 10–15 rounds to keep your heart rate elevated and metabolism active.

2. Strength-Focused Swimming

    - Use swim paddles or resistance gear to increase upper-body engagement.
    - Kickboard drills isolate the legs for a lower-body strength workout.
    - Drag workouts (swimming with a parachute or resistance band) add difficulty, similar to weightlifting.

3. Stroke Variation for Full-Body Conditioning

- Rotate strokes each lap to work different muscle groups.

- Front crawl focuses more on the upper body, while underwater running, push-offs, and kicking drills can emphasize the legs and core.

4. Treading Water for Strength & Endurance

- Perform high intensity treading (e.g., hands out of water) to challenge your core, shoulders, and legs.

- Use a dolphin kick motion or eggbeater technique to build power.

5. Add Dryland Training

- Combine swimming with bodyweight exercises (push-ups, squats, planks) for well-rounded strength.

- Stretch and perform mobility work to maintain flexibility and prevent injuries.

Part III: The Diet and Lifestyle Changes That Made the Difference

Ch 6: Nutrition Plan for Weight Loss and Blood Sugar Control

Diet Tweaks for Swimming Success

When I was suddenly diagnosed with diabetes, I knew I had to take control of my blood sugar fast. Swimming became one of my most powerful tools for managing it, but I quickly learned that what and when I ate made a huge difference in my performance and glucose levels. Thanks to my continuous glucose monitor (CGM), I was able to track patterns and fine-tune my diet for better energy, blood sugar control, and overall swimming success. These tips work well even if you aren't a diabetic!

Timing Matters: Using Swimming to Stabilize Blood Sugar

One of the biggest revelations for me was timing my swims within an hour of eating. I noticed that no matter what I ate, my blood sugar would start rising after a meal—but if I got into the pool during that window, swimming would bring it down almost instantly. This effect was rapid and consistent, making it a game-changer for my diabetes management.

If you're trying to use swimming to help control blood sugar, consider scheduling your workouts strategically:

- Swim within 30–60 minutes after eating to counteract glucose spikes.
- Monitor how different foods affect your energy and performance.
- Experiment with pre-swim snacks to find what fuels you best.

Smart Food Choices for Swimming & Blood Sugar Control

Through trial and error, I found that my body responded best to a higher-protein diet, especially when paired with balanced carbohydrates and lots of fiber. Protein provided sustained energy, helped with muscle recovery, and prevented the energy crashes I experienced when I relied too heavily on carbs alone.

Best Foods for Pre-Swim Energy & Blood Sugar Stability

Fruit + Protein – A piece of fruit (like an apple or banana) gave me quick energy but pairing it with protein helped prevent blood sugar spikes. My go-to pairings:

- Banana + cheese or almonds
- Apple + peanut butter
- Berries + Greek yogurt
- Grapes + a handful of walnuts

Lean Proteins – When I made an effort to eat more protein overall, I noticed better endurance in the pool and fewer post-workout energy crashes. Some of my best choices:

- Eggs (hard-boiled for quick snacks)
- Tuna or salmon
- Chicken or turkey
- Cottage cheese
- Protein shakes (if I was in a rush)

Hydration is Everything – One of the easiest but most crucial diet tweaks was drinking more water. Swimming may not feel like a sweaty workout, but dehydration can still sneak up on you. I made it a rule: If I thought I drank enough water, I drank one more glass!

Fine-Tuning Your Diet for Swimming Success

Everyone's body is different, but here are a few takeaways from my journey that might help you:

1. Listen to your energy levels – If I felt sluggish in the pool, I often hadn't eaten enough protein.
2. Carbs aren't the enemy – But pairing them with protein or healthy fats made a big difference in stabilizing my blood sugar.
3. Small adjustments add up – Simple changes, like hydrating better or eating protein with snacks, made my workouts more effective and my blood sugar easier to manage.

By learning how my body responded to both food and exercise, I was able to make small, sustainable diet tweaks that kept me strong in the pool and in control of my health.

Ch 7: Balancing Swimming with Other Healthy Habits

Walking and stretching for recovery

Swimming is an incredible full-body workout, but maintaining overall health goes beyond just time in the pool. I've found that incorporating walking, stretching, and quality sleep into my routine has made a huge difference in how I feel, perform, and recover. These simple but effective habits have helped me stay injury-free, maintain stable blood sugar levels, and maximize the benefits of my workouts.

Walking After Meals: A Simple Habit with Big Benefits

One of the easiest yet most effective things I do for my health is walking after every meal. If I can't make it to the pool, I make sure to get outside and walk for at least 10 minutes. This small habit has had a big impact on digestion, blood sugar stability, and overall recovery.

Why Post-Meal Walking Works

- Aids Digestion – Walking encourages faster food breakdown and nutrient absorption.
- Stabilizes Blood Sugar – A quick post-meal walk helps prevent glucose spikes by improving insulin sensitivity.
- Boosts Circulation – Movement increases blood flow to muscles and organs, reducing sluggishness.
- Supports Active Recovery – Walking keeps muscles loose and helps remove lactic acid buildup after workouts.

If you're short on time, even a 10-minute walk around the block can make a difference. The key is consistency—turn it into a daily habit!

Stretching: Essential for Injury Prevention & Performance

Stretching is one of the most overlooked but essential parts of swimming. Whether it's before an intense swim or after a tough workout, I make it a point to loosen up my muscles to avoid injury and improve flexibility.

Pre-Swim Stretching

Dynamic stretching (movement-based stretching) is best before a swim. This helps warm up muscles and increase range of motion without causing tightness. Some of my go-to stretches:

Arm Circles – Loosens up shoulders and improves mobility.

Leg Swings – Prepares hips and legs for kicking.

Torso Twists – Engages the core and improves rotation for strokes.

Post-Swim Stretching

After an intense session, I switch to static stretching (holding stretches for 20–30 seconds) to help my muscles recover. Key stretches include:

Shoulder & Triceps Stretch – Reduces tension from repetitive strokes.

Hamstring Stretch – Helps with leg flexibility and recovery.

Lower Back Stretch – Prevents tightness from core engagement during swimming.

The Power of Quality Sleep for Recovery

One of the most underrated aspects of fitness and recovery is getting enough sleep. Your body repairs and builds muscles while you rest, so if you're not sleeping well, you're not recovering properly.

Tips for Better Sleep:

Stick to a Schedule – Go to bed and wake up at the same time every day.

Limit Screens Before Bed – Blue light from phones and TVs can disrupt melatonin production.

Create a Relaxing Routine – Reading, stretching, or meditation can send a signal to your body that it's time to wind down.

Keep Your Bedroom Cool & Dark – A comfortable sleep environment makes a huge difference.

By balancing swimming with walking, stretching, and good sleep habits, you can improve recovery, prevent injuries, and keep your body performing at its best. Small, consistent habits add up over time, making it easier to maintain a healthy, active lifestyle.

The Swim Your ASS Off Challenge!

A 30-Day Commitment to a Stronger, Leaner, Healthier You

You've made it this far, and now it's time to take action! **The Swim Your ASS Off Challenge** is designed to help you burn fat, build muscle, and develop a consistent swimming habit—without burning yourself out.

This 30-day challenge is all about commitment and consistency. Instead of forcing yourself to swim every single day, the goal is to swim at least 3 days per week for the next month. This gives your body time to recover while still keeping you accountable.

How the Challenge Works

Swim at least 3 days per week – Pick the days that work best for you!

Mix up your workouts – Change your stroke, intensity, or distance to keep things fresh.

Track your progress – Keep a log of your swims, energy levels, and overall progress.

Incorporate interval training – Boost fat burning and endurance by alternating between sprints and steady swimming.

Stay hydrated and eat well – Follow the nutrition tips from this book to fuel your workouts.

Hold yourself accountable – Invite a friend to join, or share your progress online!

Your 30-Day Swim Plan

Here's a simple structured plan to guide you. Adjust as needed to fit your fitness level!

Week 1: Building the Habit

- Swim 3 days this week (easy to moderate effort, 20-30 minutes)
- Focus on form and getting comfortable in the water
- Try a mix of strokes (freestyle, backstroke, breaststroke)

Week 2: Adding Intensity

- Swim 3-4 days this week (increase duration to 30-40 minutes)
- Introduce interval training – Try 30-second sprints followed by 1-minute easy swimming
- Consider using fins or a kickboard for leg strength

Week 3: Pushing Your Limits

- Swim at least 3 days this week (aim for longer sessions – 40+ minutes)
- Test your endurance with a continuous swim goal (ex: 20+ laps)
- Add resistance – Try swimming with paddles or focus on kicking drills

Week 4: Finishing Strong

- Swim at least 3 days this week (push for max effort on one session)
- Challenge yourself to set a new personal best (speed or distance)
- End the challenge by reflecting on your progress

Bonus: Optional Cross-Training for Extra Results

- Walk or do light cardio on non-swim days to keep up activity
- Stretch or do yoga for recovery and flexibility
- Eat smart to fuel performance—protein, healthy carbs, and hydration are key!
- If you really want a challenge, incorporate some body weight or dumbbell exercises on non-swim days

Final Thoughts

By the end of these 30 days, you'll have a stronger body, a leaner and more toned physique, and a consistent fitness habit that sticks!

The goal isn't perfection—**it's commitment**. Can you complete 30 days with at least 3 swims per week?

Challenge accepted? Let's do this!

The following pages include a tracker for you to record your progress as you complete

The Swim Your ASS Off Challenge.

The Swim Your ASS Off Challenge Tracker

How to Use:

- **Mark off each swim session** on the calendar ✓.
- **Track distance & time** in the progress bar.
- **Jot down notes** about how you felt or any improvements.
- **Celebrate milestones** along the way!

Challenge Calendar:

Try to swim 3 times per week!

Week	Mon	Tue	Wed	Thu	Fri	Sat	Sun	Weekly Goal Met?
1	☐	☐	☐	☐	☐	☐	☐	☺ or ☹
2	☐	☐	☐	☐	☐	☐	☐	☺ or ☹
3	☐	☐	☐	☐	☐	☐	☐	☺ or ☹
4	☐	☐	☐	☐	☐	☐	☐	☺ or ☹
5	☐	☐						

It's ok if you don't meet your goal for a week. Try to make it up the next week!

Swim Progress Bar

Set a goal for yourself to reach by the end of the challenge (swim 20 laps, 25 minutes, or 200 meters, etc.)

Color in your progress or check them off as you complete the challenge!

Distance Goal: _____ yards/meters/laps
Time Goal: _____ minutes

Progress Chart:

☐ ☐ ☐ ☐ ☐ ☐ ☐ ☐ ☐ ☐   0% Complete
☑ ☐ ☐ ☐ ☐ ☐ ☐ ☐ ☐ ☐   10% Complete
☑ ☑ ☐ ☐ ☐ ☐ ☐ ☐ ☐ ☐   20% Complete
☑ ☑ ☑ ☐ ☐ ☐ ☐ ☐ ☐ ☐   30% Complete
☑ ☑ ☑ ☑ ☐ ☐ ☐ ☐ ☐ ☐   40% Complete
☑ ☑ ☑ ☑ ☑ ☐ ☐ ☐ ☐ ☐   50% Complete
☑ ☑ ☑ ☑ ☑ ☑ ☐ ☐ ☐ ☐   60% Complete
☑ ☑ ☑ ☑ ☑ ☑ ☑ ☐ ☐ ☐   70% Complete
☑ ☑ ☑ ☑ ☑ ☑ ☑ ☑ ☐ ☐   80% Complete
☑ ☑ ☑ ☑ ☑ ☑ ☑ ☑ ☐ ☐   90% Complete
☑ ☑ ☑ ☑ ☑ ☑ ☑ ☑ ☑ ☑   100% Complete!

Weekly Check-In

At the end of each week, reflect on your progress!

	Week 1
Wins	
Challenges	
Adjustments for Next Week	
	Week 2
Wins	
Challenges	
Adjustments for Next Week	
	Week 3
Wins	
Challenges	
Adjustments for Next Week	
	Week 4
Wins	
Challenges	
Adjustments for Next Week	
	Week 5
Wins	
Challenges	
Adjustments for Next Week	

Final Reflection:

Did you complete **The Swim Your ASS Off Challenge?**

Yes? *Not quite?*

What was your biggest improvement?

_____
_____
_____
_____

What will you do next?

_____
_____
_____
_____

Congratulations on Completing the Challenge!

Whether you crushed every swim session or simply made progress toward your goals, you've taken a huge step in building strength, endurance, and a healthier lifestyle. Keep the momentum going—set new challenges, explore different swim workouts, and most importantly, have fun in the water. This is just the beginning!

www.ingramcontent.com/pod-product-compliance
Lightning Source LLC
Chambersburg PA
CBHW070547030426
42337CB00016B/2382